You can quit OVERTHINKING

A book guide to stopping over contemplations

Kenneth Furrow

Copyright © by Kenneth Furrow

2024.

transferred, nor kept in a database. Neither in Part nor full can the document be copied, scanned, faxed, or retained without approval from the publisher or creator.

TABLE OF CONTENTS

Knowing the difference between overthinking and productive thinking

Detecting Triggers

Acknowledging circumstances and feelings that lead to excessive pondering

Techniques to help you become more conscious of your mental processes

Rewire your mental processes

Cognitive strategies to alter unfavorable thought habits

The significance of mental changes and affirmations that are good

Introduction

With 'You Can Quit Overthinking", we set out on a life-changing path to recover the clarity and tranquility that overthinking has stolen from us. This book is more than just a list of techniques; it is a lifesaver for those who feel trapped by their own ideas and a manual for handling mental turmoil with poise and fortitude.

Fundamentally, this book recognizes that overanalyzing complicates our lives in addition to making decisions more difficult. We provide the foundation for significant mental transformations with a well-chosen examination of the nature of overthinking, the factors that set off cycles of excessive contemplation, and the difference between constructive and harmful thought processes.

With its insights about rewiring mental processes, stress management, embracing mindfulness, and building a supportive network, each chapter represents a step towards liberation. You Can Quit Overthinking is a plan for a more conscious, contented life rather than just a guide for controlling thoughts.

This book is proof of the ability for transformation that exists inside every one of us. It serves as a reminder that we can shift our focus from overanalyzing to living completely in the present moment if we have the correct knowledge and tools. Greetings from the start of your journey towards a life in which your ideas work as allies rather than as enemies.

Chapter 1

Comprehending Overthinking

A maze of excessive, frequently negative ideas and overthinking can trap the mind and have a major detrimental effect on one's quality of life. It is a widespread problem that cuts across age, gender, and background. It shows itself as never-ending cycles of dwelling on the past, worrying about the future, and generally overanalyzing life's little moments. This mental behavior can have numerous negative psychological and physical repercussions that impair one's general health and capacity to carry out everyday tasks.

The excessive amount of ideas that are primarily pessimistic or focused on the future is what distinguishes overthinking from other types of thinking. People who are enmeshed in a web of overthinking frequently find themselves engaged in a loop of worry and anxiety, which can result in serious emotional suffering. The consequences of this might be extensive, impacting not only one's bodily but also mental health. Overthinkers frequently report experiencing symptoms like headaches, stomach problems, and sleep disruptions, underscoring the concrete effects of this abstract disorder.

Overanalyzing can also result in a decline in creativity and productivity. A person's mental capacity for problem-solving, creative reasoning, and decision-making is reduced when they are consumed by negative ideas or fictitious situations. This can impede both professional and personal development since chances for advancement may be lost owing to uncertainty or hesitation brought on by overly critical thinking.

Relationships can be strained by overthinking. The propensity to interpret events or discussions too broadly can result in miscommunications and disputes, which exacerbate feelings of loneliness or isolation. This social disengagement may set off a vicious cycle in which an absence of encouraging relationships fuels an increase in overthinking and vice versa.

Overanalyzing Is a Common Issue. It is impossible to exaggerate how common overthinking is in contemporary culture. It makes sense that many people are suffering from overanalysis given the constant barrage of information and the pressure to live up to social norms.

Although this conduct is frequently an ineffective attempt at self-defense or problem-solving, it can be harmful to one's pleasure and health.

Overthinking's physical effects, such as elevated stress levels, can cause major health problems, like heart difficulties. Excessive rumination can cause a stress reaction that increases heart rate and blood pressure, further taxing the heart. Moreover, disruptions to eating and sleeping schedules can impair the body's capacity to heal and remain in a healthy state, which can weaken the immune system and make a person more susceptible to disease.

There is a substantial correlation between overthinking and mental health illnesses like anxiety, sadness, and PTSD, which raises concerns about the psychological implications of overthinking.

Constant mental stress can change how the brain functions, impacting mood control, decision-making, and concentration. This may result in a vicious cycle when mental health problems are made worse by overthinking, which then fuels the cycle of overthinking.

It's critical to recognize the difference between overthinking and useful thinking. Goal-oriented, solution-focused, and yielding practical insights are the hallmarks of productive thinking. It entails a methodical approach to problem-solving, where ideas are arranged to help one reach a particular goal. This way of thinking promotes effectiveness, efficiency, and creative problem-solving. It is distinguished by clarity, direction, and purpose.

On the other hand, overthinking is characterized by a lack of progress, in which ideas recur without coming up with a solution. This can result in analysis paralysis, wherein the inability to make any decisions at all is due to the dread of choosing the incorrect choice. Overanalyzing, in contrast to productive thinking, is stressful, depletes mental resources, and frequently has unfavorable effects.

To control overthinking, one must grasp how these two ways of thinking differ from each other. People can use techniques to refocus their attention on more constructive and positive thought patterns by identifying when their thoughts are deviating into unproductive areas. This change is essential for ending the overthinking loop and achieving a more balanced, healthy mental state.

The characteristics of excessive thinking and how it affects our existence

Overanalyzing is a widespread problem that many people experience. It is an overabundance of thinking, usually with an emphasis on the negative or worries about the future. This behavior can have a negative effect on one's bodily and emotional well-being and result in a number of issues.

Although overthinking is not a recognized medical word, there is ample evidence of its detrimental impacts on well-being. Overthinkers frequently dwell on unfavorable ideas, revisit unpleasant memories, and worry about what might happen in the future. This pattern has the potential to worsen and impair daily functioning and thought processes. Overanalyzing crosses the line into a problem area when it starts to negatively impact sleep, eating, or social interactions. It is interesting to note that some people overthink things in an attempt to protect themselves, presuming that bad things happen in order to protect themselves from disappointments or injuries.

Overthinking has bodily consequences in addition to mental ones. Headaches, tummy issues, and accompanying anxiety are common symptoms in people who suffer from overthinking. This is due to the fact that overthinking-related stress and anxiety can have a physical manifestation and impact different body systems. Excessive stress brought on by overanalyzing might raise blood pressure and increase the risk of heart-related problems, including heart attacks or strokes. Stress can also result in bad behaviors like smoking or binge drinking, which puts one's physical health at further risk.

Sleep and hunger are two areas where overthinking affects people negatively. An inability to stop thinking can cause serious sleep disturbances that can lead to insomnia or poor-quality sleep. This has an impact on general health, mood, and productivity during the day. In a similar vein, overanalyzing can suppress or interfere with regular eating habits, which can result in overeating or appetite loss, both of which are detrimental to one's health.

There is a strong correlation between overthinking and mental health conditions such as anxiety, sadness, PTSD, and borderline personality disorder. It can change the structure and connectivity of the brain, resulting in mood disorders and impairing concentration, problem-solving, and decision-making skills. Overthinking causes continual stress, which impairs immunity and increases susceptibility to illnesses and infections.

Even though overthinking can seem like an unstoppable force, it can be managed with certain techniques. Identification of triggers is an essential initial step. Focus can be diverted from unfavorable ideas by using strategies like journaling, focused activities, and regulated breathing exercises. Creating a strong social network and getting expert assistance is also crucial if overanalyzing affects someone's life negatively.

Overthinking is a widespread problem that can have a serious impact on someone's physical and mental well-being. People can lessen its effects and enhance their quality of life by being aware of its nature and effects and using management techniques.

Knowing the difference between overthinking and productive thinking

A constructive approach that produces useful insights or solutions is called productive thinking. It is distinguished by a targeted and goal-oriented approach to planning and problem-solving.

Productive thinkers follow a methodical cognitive process in which ideas and steps are built upon to produce a cohesive understanding or course of action. This kind of thought is characterized by direction, clarity, and purpose. It frequently entails establishing clear goals, investigating several possibilities, assessing advantages and disadvantages, and coming to judgments based on information or insights that are already available. Time is not a constraint on productive thinking; rather, it is determined by the caliber and usefulness of one's ideas in reaching a goal.

When planning a project, for example, productive thinking might entail determining the project's objectives, outlining the procedures required to reach those objectives, spotting potential roadblocks and finding workarounds, and wisely allocating resources. The thinker keeps the final result in mind at all times, making sure that every choice they make and every idea they have helps them get there. Efficiency, inventiveness, and creativity are all nourished by productive thought. It makes it possible for people to approach problems with an eye toward finding answers, which promotes efficient problem-solving and decision-making.

On the other hand, overthinking is a counterproductive mental process that results in excessive rumination on a specific subject, circumstance, or choice without producing any useful results. Overthinkers frequently get stuck in a cycle of looping ideas, going over the same problems over and over again without moving forward or coming to a decision. This kind of thinking results in delay and indecision because it is motivated by fear, anxiety, or uncertainty. Perfectionism, overbearing duty, or the dread of making the incorrect choice can all be causes of overthinking.

An overthinker could, for instance, become fixated on every scenario when making a decision to change careers, constantly doubting if it's the right choice, what might go wrong, and whether they have taken all relevant variables into account. Making decisions is paralyzed by this never-ending loop of analysis, which keeps the person from moving forward in any meaningful way. Overanalyzing depletes mental reserves, raises stress and anxiety levels, and can have a detrimental effect on general well-being. Overthinking, in contrast to effective thinking, results in mental stagnation and unhappiness rather than answers or positive outcomes.

Thus, overthinking is an unproductive cycle of rumination that results in delay, indecision, and increased stress, whereas productive thinking is an organized, goal-oriented process that yields practical insights and solutions.

It is essential to understand the distinction between these two ways of thinking in order to solve problems effectively and preserve mental health.

Chapter 2

Detecting Triggers

When it comes to overthinking, figuring out what sets off this exhausting mental loop is like trying to discover a map in a maze. It's important to comprehend both the internal feelings that cause us to go into an unending cycle of thought as well as the exterior events that occur. The goal of this detecting journey is to weave through the complex web of our experiences and responses, not to tick things off a list.

Uncertainty and change are often the breeding grounds for overthinking. Unpredictable events in life, including taking on new challenges or venturing into uncharted territory, can cause a mental storm. Not the shift per se, but the uncertainty and powerlessness it entails frequently send us down a path of undue reflection.

In a similar vein, critical decision-making situations serve as triggers for overanalyzing. Whether they are made in our personal or professional lives, the weight of these choices can paralyze us in terror. Fear of making the incorrect decision traps us in a never-ending cycle of thought and keeps us from acting at all.

Overanalyzing can also develop from social interactions. We often repeat conversations and situations in our minds long after they have ended because we are afraid of being perceived negatively, afraid of saying the wrong thing, or afraid of losing someone's favor.

Overthinking is also greatly influenced by our past experiences. Anxiety and caution might influence our actions in the present and future due to recollections of past mistakes, traumatic occurrences, or even small inaccuracies. We frequently get stuck in our past thinking, unable to go forward.

Comparing ourselves to other people in the digital era, particularly via social media, can make overthinking worse. This never-ending comparison of our lives to others' highlights can leave us feeling dissatisfied and driven to change our situation no matter what.

The emotional terrain that encourages overanalyzing is wide-ranging and complex. For example, fear and anxiety are the main forces behind a vicious cycle of concern that reinforces itself. Our confidence and judgment can be undermined by insecurity and self-doubt, which makes us second-guess every action and idea.   Depression and hopelessness can cause us to become fixated on our circumstances, previous decisions, and future, which exacerbates our sense of helplessness. While remorse and regret can keep us stuck in a loop of "what ifs"and "if onlys,"anger and irritation can cause us to get fixated on injustices or disappointments.

Overthinking can be triggered by a variety of factors, and addressing them requires a multifaceted strategy that incorporates cognitive behavioral therapy, emotional regulation, and mindfulness. It's about finding healthy ways to handle emotions, questioning illogical notions, and remaining in the moment. Help from loved ones, friends, or mental health specialists can also offer direction and useful methods for effectively controlling overthinking.

Essentially, identifying triggers involves comprehending the intricate relationship that exists between our internal feelings and our environment. It's a self-discovery journey that calls for tolerance, empathy, and a readiness to face and make sense of the maze that is our minds.

Acknowledging circumstances and feelings that lead to excessive pondering

A prevalent mental habit that can cause worries, tension, and lost opportunities is overthinking. Rather than coming up with answers or moving forward with constructive action, it frequently entails moping over issues, second-guessing choices, and conjuring up worst-case scenarios. Managing this habit and promoting a healthier mental state requires an understanding of the circumstances and feelings that set off overthinking.

Circumstances That Lead to Overthinking:

1. Uncertainty and Change: Overthinking can occur in the circumstances involving uncertainty

or major changes, such as relocating to a new city, beginning a new job, or dealing with unforeseen circumstances. These circumstances' lack of control and predictability can cause excessive concern about possible outcomes.

2. High-Stakes judgments: Overanalyzing is frequently the result of making judgments that carry a lot of weight, both personally and professionally. People who are afraid of making the incorrect decision may

become paralyzed by their own thinking.

3. Social Interactions: Overanalyzing can occur in social circumstances, especially when there are new or unfamiliar persons involved. Overthinking social interactions and exchanges can result from worries about being perceived negatively, saying the incorrect thing, or losing someone's favor.

4. Past Experiences: Stressful or unfavorable past events can cause overthinking in comparable present-

day or future circumstances. This might involve everything from painful experiences to prior mistakes, where the recollection causes anxiety and overly cautious behavior.

5. Comparison with Others: Making comparisons with others, particularly on social media, can lead to excessive reflection on one's own decisions, accomplishments, and values. This frequently results in discontent and excessive contemplation of how to make one's circumstances better or different.

Feelings That Lead to Overthinking:

1. Anxiety and Fear: The two main emotions that lead to overthinking are anxiety and fear. The mind creates a vicious cycle of anxiety by continuously considering what can go wrong in an attempt to foresee and prevent unfavorable consequences.

2. Insecurity and Self-Doubt: These emotions might cause someone to overanalyze their worth, skills, and judgment. This frequently leads to ongoing introspection and reflection,

which undermines confidence and impairs judgment.

3. melancholy and despair: People who are experiencing melancholy or despair may find themselves obsessing over their circumstances, choices from the past, and hopes for the future. This can make one feel even more forlorn and discourage them from acting to make their circumstances or mood better.

4. Anger and Frustration: Anger and frustration can lead to overthinking, particularly when people focus on

what made them angry, how they might respond to the circumstance, or how they might prevent it from happening again.

5. Guilt and Regret: Thinking too much about what could have been done differently can be a result of feeling guilty or regretful about past decisions. This frequently entails thinking through alternative scenarios and repeating events.

Handling Triggers of Overthinking: Identifying the circumstances and feelings that lead to overthinking is the first step in controlling this behavior. Once overthinking has been recognized, people can address and lessen it with approaches including mindfulness, cognitive-behavioral techniques, and emotional control skills. These tactics consist of being in the present moment, confronting unreasonable ideas, and coming up with healthy methods to handle emotions. Moreover, getting help from loved ones, friends, or mental health specialists can offer direction and practical overthinking management techniques.

Techniques to help you become more conscious of your mental processes

You can use a variety of successful ways to become more aware of and modify your thought habits. These solutions draw on psychological concepts, mindfulness practices, and cognitive-behavioral procedures. Implementing these tactics will take time and effort, but they can dramatically improve your mental health and life pleasure.

1. discipline Mindfulness and Meditation: Mindfulness is the discipline of becoming completely present and engaged in the present moment without judgment. Mindfulness helps you become more aware of your thoughts, feelings, and bodily sensations as they arise. Meditation, a practice commonly used to increase mindfulness, can help you examine your thinking

patterns without becoming engrossed in them. Regular mindfulness meditation can raise your awareness of negative thought patterns and provide you the opportunity to choose how to respond to them mindfully rather than reactively.

2. Keep a Thought Log: Writing down your ideas can be an effective approach to becoming more conscious of your thought patterns, particularly those that are negative or unproductive. When you catch yourself indulging in negative

thinking, write down the thought, the trigger, and how you felt afterward. Over time, examining your thought diary can help you uncover patterns and triggers for negative thinking, which is the first step toward changing them.

3. Challenge and recast Negative Thoughts: Once you've become aware of your negative thought patterns, question their correctness and recast them in a more positive or realistic context. This entails challenging the data supporting your negative views,

exploring alternate interpretations, and focusing on solutions rather than problems. For example, if you have a tendency to make generalizations based on a single unpleasant experience, remind yourself that one event does not determine future outcomes. This cognitive reorganization can help you achieve a more balanced and optimistic view.

4. Practice Expressive Writing: Expressing yourself via writing can help you understand and make sense of your thoughts, feelings, and

experiences. This can be especially useful for breaking out from troublesome or persistent mental habits. Set aside time every day to write in a notebook, exploring your innermost feelings without judgment. Over time, this practice can help you acquire insight into your thought patterns and cultivate a more aware and compassionate relationship with yourself.

5. Conduct Behavioral Experiments: To question and change your thought habits, consider evaluating the

validity of your negative views using behavioral experiments. For example, if you are afraid that making a mistake may have disastrous consequences, consciously allow yourself to make little mistakes in a controlled environment and observe the results. Often, the outcomes are less bad than you expected, which might help diminish the power of catastrophic thinking.

6. Surround Yourself with Positive Influences: The people around you have a huge impact on your mental

patterns. Surround yourself with people who are helpful, encouraging, and self-aware. They will urge you to think constructively. Engaging with people who demonstrate good thinking and conduct can motivate you to follow suit in your own life.

7. Seek expert Help: If you are having difficulty becoming aware of or changing your thought patterns on your own, consider obtaining assistance from a mental health expert. Cognitive-behavioral therapy (CBT) and other therapeutic

treatments can provide systematic direction for recognizing, confronting, and changing negative thought patterns.

Implementing these tactics necessitates continual effort and self-compassion. Remember that altering deeply ingrained mental habits takes time. Celebrate your accomplishments along the journey, and be kind to yourself when you face setbacks.

Even though she was a seasoned project manager, Anna

couldn't stop thinking about the outcomes of her decisions, which caused her to lose sleep and work less efficiently. The concept of maintaining a thought diary, which she picked up in a mindfulness workshop, was the catalyst for her turning point. By keeping track of the thoughts and feelings that caused her to overanalyze, Anna was able to identify her perfectionist streak and fear of failure as key factors. She was able to cut down on her overthinking since she was self-aware enough to face these emotions head-on. She noticed an improvement in both her mental health and the morale and productivity of her staff when she started establishing more reasonable expectations for everyone.

Chapter 3

Rewire your mental processes

It takes more than just blocking out the negative voices in our heads to change the way we think. We need to reframe those bad thoughts into forces that drive us forward. This approach, which is firmly based on cognitive-behavioral therapy (CBT) principles, transforms us from being our own worst enemies into our greatest allies. It is open to anybody who is ready to set out on this road of self-awareness and transformation.

The cognitive restructuring technique is at the core of this change. Think of your thoughts as a garden. The bright blooms of your good ideas have been overshadowed by the negative thoughts that have grown like weeds over time. The gardening tool you use to cultivate a more pleasant mental environment and remove these detrimental thoughts is called cognitive restructuring.

The first step in the process is self-monitoring, which is similar to observing which plants are flourishing and which are being suffocated by weeds when strolling around your garden. It's important to be conscious of the negative thought patterns that have gotten so ingrained in daily life that they are nearly invisible. Writing in a notebook serves as a gardening journal where you record the ideas, feelings, and situations that set off these patterns.

Next, consider the underlying presumptions of these ideas. It's similar to attentively inspecting weeds and discovering they are not as firmly established as you formerly believed. You are making space for fresh ideas to be sown by questioning these presumptions.

The second stage is to gather evidence, which is similar to choosing the correct seeds for your garden. This entails seeking out instances and data that refute your pessimistic beliefs and demonstrate that they are not entirely accurate. It's about seeing the abundance of opportunities that lie outside of your existing frame of reference by widening your perspective.

You begin to develop fresh thoughts when you come up with replacements. These are the ideas that are more realistic, upbeat, and balanced. It involves using your imagination to conjure up alternative scenarios and viewpoints that are more in line with the garden you wish to create.

This mental gardening has many significant effects. A revitalized sense of self-confidence, better relationships, and less stress and anxiety are just a few of the flowers that will start to emerge. It's a metamorphosis that improves every aspect of your life and alters the terrain of your thoughts.

While it is possible to go through this process alone, consulting with a therapist can offer the direction and encouragement needed to get through it successfully. They are similar to the knowledgeable gardeners who can assist you with weed identification, seed selection, and full-flower gardening.

Your new garden needs sunshine and water to thrive, and these can be found in positive affirmations and mental adjustments. Positive affirmations serve as daily nourishment, serving as a constant reminder of your value, potential, and the goals you have set for yourself.

They are the act of introducing truth and kindness into your life, encouraging the development of your new mental terrain.

Changes in perspective that enable you to view obstacles as chances for personal development, setbacks as learning experiences, and uncertainty as a route toward exploration are known as mindset shifts. It's a change from a fixed perspective—where challenges are perceived as threats—to a growth mindset, where challenges are seen as opportunities to grow and change.

Including these routines, such as visualizing your goals or saying affirmations in the morning, into your everyday routine helps to cement the improvements you're making. It all comes down to repetition, consistency, and a sincere belief in the transformational potential of these activities.

The efficacy of these methods is supported by science. Reward centers in the brain are activated by positive affirmations and mindset modifications, which strengthen positive self-perception and an optimistic outlook.

Rewiring your brain is essentially about creating a mental garden where optimistic ideas thrive. A more contented, robust, and serene life is the reward for the voyage, which calls for endurance, patience, and care.

*Cognitive strategies to alter
unfavorable thought habits*

Cognitive approaches for modifying negative thinking patterns entail a methodical strategy to recognize, question, and alter harmful thoughts that contribute to emotional suffering and mental health difficulties. These strategies are important to cognitive restructuring, a core component of cognitive-behavioral therapy (CBT), aiming at deconstructing problematic concepts and recreating them in a more balanced and correct way. Some of the strategies for Cognitive Restructuring include:

Self-Monitoring: The basis of changing negative thought patterns is acknowledging those thoughts. Self-monitoring entails being aware of your thoughts, especially those that precede or accompany painful experiences. Journaling is a recommended strategy for monitoring thoughts, emotions, and the conditions in which they occur, helping to detect patterns and triggers of negative thinking.

Questioning Assumptions: After identifying negative beliefs, the next stage is to examine their veracity. This includes reviewing the evidence for and against these views, recognizing cognitive distortions, and determining whether these thoughts are founded on facts or biased perceptions.

Gathering Evidence: Central to cognitive restructuring is the collection of evidence that supports or contradicts your negative views. This process entails critically examining situations, seeking evidence that challenges erroneous or unreasonable views, and contemplating alternate explanations for events.

Generating Alternatives: Developing alternative, more positive, or balanced thinking is vital for changing harmful patterns. This could involve exploring multiple viewpoints on an issue, making positive affirmations, or evaluating realistic possibilities rather than worst-case scenarios.

Benefits of Cognitive Restructuring: Learning to identify and modify negative thought patterns has various benefits, including less stress and anxiety, greater communication skills, healthier relationships, replacement of unhealthy coping mechanisms, and the rebuilding of self-confidence and self-esteem. These improvements can considerably enhance overall well-being and life satisfaction.

Application and Effectiveness

While cognitive restructuring techniques can be done individually, engaging with a therapist, particularly one skilled in CBT, can give essential advice and support. A therapist can help with detecting cognitive distortions, comprehending the irrationality of particular views, and practicing restructuring procedures effectively. Over time, individuals can learn to apply these tactics independently, helping them to regulate negative thoughts more effectively when they come.

Cognitive restructuring has been demonstrated to be useful for a range of mental health illnesses, including anxiety, depression, and PTSD, as well as in handling hard life transitions and relationship issues. It gives a practical strategy for changing the way we think, ultimately impacting how we feel and act in a positive manner.

Cognitive strategies for modifying negative thought patterns are effective tools within cognitive-behavioral therapy that help individuals confront and transform destructive thoughts. By adopting these approaches, individuals can develop more mental calm, resilience, and a more optimistic attitude toward life, contributing to enhanced mental health and well-being.

The significance of mental changes and affirmations that are good

The merging of positive affirmations and mindset shifts gives a solid method for countering the often devastating habit of overthinking. This thorough content dives into their value, backed by psychological theories and empirical facts, providing a full grasp of how these practices can improve mental health and well-being.

Understanding Positive Affirmations

Positive affirmations are present-tense comments that represent one's desired state of being or aims. They are intended to be empowering, affirming beliefs and values that are significant to the individual. By constantly repeating these affirmations, one can rewire the subconscious mind, developing a happy mindset and attracting wonderful experiences into one's life.

The Benefits of Positive Affirmations

- Boosts Self-Confidence: Affirmations assist in overcoming self-doubt and developing a strong sense of self-worth and confidence in one's talents, therefore enabling a positive response to obstacles.

- Enhances Focus and Clarity: They direct attention toward objectives and aspirations, improving motivation and clarity, thereby laying the stage for achievement.

- Reduces Stress and Anxiety: Replacing negative ideas with good ones through affirmations can dramatically reduce stress and promote inner calm.

- Attracts Positivity and Abundance: According to the law of attraction, positive ideas and beliefs attract favorable events, cultivating a mindset that is receptive to receiving positivity.

Mindset Shifts to Stop Overthinking

Overthinking can be a direct result of a stuck attitude when obstacles are regarded as threats rather than chances for progress. Shifting to a growth mindset, where one perceives obstacles as chances to learn and better, can greatly reduce overthinking. This change emphasizes embracing uncertainty and viewing failures as stepping stones, building resilience and a proactive approach towards life adversities.

Implementing Positive Affirmations and Mindset Shifts

-Morning Affirmation Practice: Begin your day by acknowledging your talents and aspirations. Find a quiet area, utilize a mirror, and boldly recite your affirmations aloud, internalizing their good words.

- vision: Pair affirmations with vision, imagining the successful realization of your goals while you affirm. Engage all senses to improve the emotional connection with your affirmations.

- Consistency and Repetition: Make affirmations a daily practice. Consistency is crucial to integrating these positive phrases into your subconscious, gradually influencing your thinking.

The Science Behind Positive Affirmations

The psychological theory of self-affirmation states that affirmations assist in sustaining our feelings of self-integrity by affirming our views in positive ways. This practice is substantiated by neuroscientific research, suggesting that self-affirmations activate brain areas connected with self-related processing and reward, reinforcing positive self-perception and future orientation.

The practice of positive affirmations, paired with a move towards a development mindset, is a potent technique for breaking the cycle of overthinking. By establishing a positive mindset, improving self-confidence, and embracing adversities as chances for progress, individuals can dramatically improve their mental well-being and general quality of life. Embracing these disciplines involves intention, consistency, and conviction in their transformational power, leading to a more full and happier life.

Michael, a software developer, struggled with negative self-talk and catastrophic predictions, especially while facing tough coding problems. His breakthrough occurred when he accepted cognitive-behavioral therapy (CBT) practices. Michael learned to identify illogical thoughts and replace them with more balanced, positive affirmations. For instance, instead of thinking, "I'll never solve this problem,"he would remind himself, "I've solved similar problems before, and I can figure this out too."This transformation in perspective led to a tremendous improvement in his problem-solving skills and confidence. Michael's experience demonstrates the ability to rewire mental processes to combat overthinking.

Chapter 4

The De-Stress Formula

Stress is a typical enemy in the dynamic field of web development, where the digital landscape is always changing and there is constant pressure to create creative solutions. You are no stranger to the difficulties that arise when trying to strike a balance between the demands of your job and your own mental and physical health as a web developer. This story explores the life-changing experience of Jane, a high school teacher who learned to use "The De-stress Formula" to help her manage the challenges in both her personal and professional lives.

The unrelenting speed of Jane's schedule and the continual juggling act between her career and personal obligations left the committed educator feeling overburdened. She could feel the tension permeating every part of her life, including her relationships with the pupils and her alone time. She felt exhausted and cut off from the core of teaching, which was something she loved, during this period when the cycle of overthinking threatened to overwhelm her.

Jane sought to incorporate mindfulness and relaxation techniques into her daily routine as a means of finding a solution. She started with basic yet effective techniques like deep breathing exercises and meditation, which she discovered to be a haven from the chaos of her thoughts. Even while these exercises were scary at first, they eventually became a part of her routine and gave her a break from her mind's constant chatter.

Jane, too, accepted the benefit of diversion and took comfort in her favorite pastimes. These activities, which included taking up new hobbies or volunteering at a nearby charity, provided a reminder that life was more than simply stress and work. They served as an example of the wonders of being in the moment and appreciating the small things in life.

As Jane learned more about mindfulness, she came to understand the transformational potential of self-compassion exercises. She developed a constructive self-talk pattern that changed her viewpoint from one of criticism to one of kindness by learning to accept her thoughts and feelings without passing judgment. This change was more than simply a mental workout; it was a fundamental adjustment to her way of living that gave her the fortitude she needed to face the difficulties she faced at work.

For Jane, journaling her ideas became a therapeutic activity that gave her a platform to express her emotions and spot trends that led to her overanalysis. Her perspective and clarity were restored when she combined this practice with the mindfulness methods she had chosen.

Jane faced difficulties on her voyage. There were times when she felt anxiety and doubt and that the burden of her obligations was too much to bear. However, Jane found her strength during these exposed moments. She discovered how to see her challenges as chances for development and resiliency rather than as failures.

Jane's life had taken a surprising turn. She reported a considerable reduction in her stress levels and an increase in her presence and engagement when interacting with pupils. She had a fresh appreciation for life's small pleasures, hence her love for teaching was reignited. Jane's tale is a powerful example of the value of maintaining equilibrium in the face of hardship and the strength of resilience.

By using "The De-stress Formula"in her day-to-day activities, Jane found a comprehensive method for stress management and avoided overthinking. This method benefited her productivity and quality of life as a web developer. Her experience serves as a reminder that resilience is about more than just conquering obstacles; it's also about developing strength while doing so.

Jane's tale offers hope to people who are stuck in a stressful loop of overanalyzing things. It serves as an example of how self-compassion, mindfulness, and relaxation techniques may change how one approaches life and work. Through the implementation of "The De-stress Formula,"Jane was able to effectively handle her stress, avoid overanalyzing situations, and eventually improve her overall well-being and output. Her story is an example to everyone who wants to face the challenges of contemporary life with grace and resiliency.

Stress management methods that prevent overthinking

1. Find a Distraction:

Engaging in things that you enjoy might be an effective approach to shut down overthinking. Taking up a new pastime, learning new kitchen skills, attending your favorite gym class, or volunteering with a local charity might divert your focus from stress-inducing ideas to something more positive and constructive. If beginning something new feels scary, consider committing a fixed amount of time, such as 30 minutes every other day, to explore possible distractions or participate in existing ones. This strategy can help stop the cycle of overthinking by busying your mind with tasks that need focus and ingenuity.

2. Deep Breathing Techniques:

Deep breathing is a well-documented approach for relieving stress and anxiety. A simple exercise entails finding a comfortable location to sit, relaxing your neck and shoulders, placing one palm on your heart and the other on your abdomen, and then breathing and exhaling through your nose. This concentrates your attention on the physical sensations of breathing, helping to quiet your mind and lessen racing thoughts. Practicing this practice for just 5 minutes, three times a day, or whenever you feel overwhelmed by overthinking, can bring immediate relief.

3. Meditation

Regular meditation practice is a wonderful technique for cleansing your mind of nervous chatter and focusing your attention. It assists in lowering stress and increasing your general mental well-being by generating a feeling of relaxation and presence. You can start with easy mindfulness exercises, focusing on your breath and gradually bringing your attention back whenever your mind wanders. This exercise can be particularly good for those who find themselves constantly stuck in cycles of overthinking, offering an opportunity to reset and calm the mind.

4. Practicing Mindfulness and Staying Present:

Mindfulness includes grounding yourself in the present moment, which may be immensely beneficial in managing overthinking. Simple habits like unplugging from digital gadgets, eating mindfully, or taking a walk outside and focusing on your environment can help divert your attention away from unpleasant thoughts. These activities enable you to appreciate the moment, lessening the inclination to concentrate on previous mistakes or worry about future outcomes.

5. Consider Other Viewpoints: Overthinking entails fixating on a single perspective, usually anticipating bad outcomes. By actively exploring different opinions

and questioning the truth of your anxious beliefs, you can get a more balanced perspective.

Writing down your views and critically examining their correctness can help break down the loop of negative thinking and open up new, more optimistic ways of perceiving events.

6. Practice Self-Compassion: Self-criticism can fuel overthinking, especially when ruminating on previous actions or imagined mistakes.

Practicing self-compassion entails noticing and embracing your feelings without judgment. Adopting supportive self-talk, such as I am doing my best or I am enough, can help alter your mindset from one of criticism to one of kindness and understanding towards oneself. This method helps lessen the tension associated with overthinking by cultivating a more forgiving and sympathetic attitude toward your own experiences.

7. Write Down Your Thoughts: Writing down your thoughts and feelings helps bring clarity and minimize the intensity of overthinking. By externalizing your issues, you may find that they hold less influence over you, making it easier to let go of unnecessary worry. After writing, allow yourself some time away from these thoughts, such as a 24-hour period, to get perspective and prevent impulsive behaviors that can increase stress. This technique can also aid in detecting patterns in

your thoughts that may contribute to overthinking, allowing for more constructive methods to approach stress.

Implementing these approaches can help manage and lessen the stress associated with overthinking. By actively engaging in distraction, deep breathing, meditation, mindfulness, considering other viewpoints, practicing self-compassion, and writing down your thoughts, you can develop a more balanced and healthier approach to managing stress and preventing overthinking from diminishing your quality of life.

Combining mindfulness and relaxation techniques to everyday living

Incorporating relaxation and mindfulness techniques into daily life can serve as an effective de-stress formula, improving general well-being and enhancing one's quality of life. This comprehensive method involves knowing the basics of mindfulness, recognizing the benefits of such practices, and adopting strategies that can be seamlessly integrated into daily routines.

Understanding Mindfulness and its Benefits

Mindfulness is the practice of being fully present in the moment and aware of your thoughts and feelings without distraction or judgment. This simple yet profound practice has roots in meditation and has been linked to a myriad of health benefits, including enhanced cognitive flexibility, improved emotion regulation, greater empathy, and better focus and attention.

Additionally, mindfulness techniques have been found to support diabetes control, bolster the immune system response, improve memory, foster positive emotions and relationships, encourage relaxation, and elevate self-compassion and self-esteem.

Practical Strategies for Daily Integration

1. Intentional Breathing Exercises

Intentional breathing is a cornerstone of mindfulness that can greatly reduce stress. Techniques like the 4-7-8 breath, created by Andrew Weil, are based on yoga principles and are meant to induce relaxation. By focusing on your breath, you activate the parasympathetic nervous system, which starts a relaxation response, lowering heart rate, blood pressure, and respiration.

2. Mindful Movement

Incorporating mindful movement into your daily life, such as yoga, tai chi, or even mindful walking, can significantly improve stress management. These practices combine rhythmic breathing with a number of postures or movements, improving physical health while also centering the mind.

3. Guided Imagery and Meditation

Guided imagery and meditation can be strong tools for relaxation and stress reduction. Using audio guides for practices like body scans, mindful standing yoga, or mindfulness meditation on breath, sounds, thoughts, and feelings can help relax the body and mind. These techniques do not require any special equipment and can be performed anywhere, making them easily accessible.

4. Daily Mindfulness Habits

Integrate mindfulness into daily tasks through easy actions like mindful eating, paying attention to the sensations of each bite, or practicing mindfulness while performing daily chores, such as washing dishes or walking. These moments provide chances to cultivate awareness and presence.

5. Mindful Use of Technology

Setting boundaries around technology use can also promote mindfulness. Dedicate specific times for checking emails or social media, and use technology actively rather than as a default activity. This helps keep focus and reduces the stress linked with constant connectivity.

6. Creating Mindfulness Prompts

Establish habits or prompts that remind you to practice mindfulness throughout the day. This could be a set time for meditation, a journal for capturing morning thoughts, or a visual reminder in your office. These ideas can help reinforce your mindfulness practice and make it a regular part of your day.

Incorporating relaxation and mindfulness practices into daily life offers a holistic approach to managing stress and improving well-being. By understanding the benefits of mindfulness and adopting practical strategies for daily integration, people can improve their mental, emotional, and physical health. The key to successful mindfulness practice lies in

consistency and finding the right mix of methods that fit into your lifestyle.

Chapter 5

Manage Your Resources and Time

A straightforward yet effective method for dealing with stress, anxiety, and the emotional fallout from traumatic experiences is expressive writing. This approach, which is based on writing down one's thoughts and emotions, is a therapeutic tool that helps people make sense of the complex emotional landscapes they find themselves in.

The core of expressive writing is its capacity to promote self-awareness, facilitate emotional release, and develop coping mechanisms that improve mental health.

Journaling is not the same as expressive writing. It's a deliberate, targeted practice that explores the complexities of one's emotional experiences, providing a special path for introspection and emotional release. This can be especially helpful for people who are struggling with anxiety, stress, or the aftereffects of traumatic events. People can gain an understanding of their stressors and anxiety triggers by putting their thoughts and emotions on paper. This opens the door to cognitive restructuring and emotional healing.

Exposing the Emotional Layers

The revealing of emotions is the central idea of expressive writing. People can make meaning of their emotions through this process, which gives them a sense of empowerment and control. For example, John, a college student suffering from severe exam anxiety, turned to expressive writing for comfort and comprehension. Through the process of recording his worries and stresses, John was able to analyze his anxiety, pinpoint its origins, and create useful coping strategies.

People can question and change harmful thought habits through this transformative process, which greatly lessens stress and anxiety symptoms. Reflective writing allows one to identify and change the

stories that feed worry, substituting more realistic and helpful viewpoints.
Fostering Emotional Hardiness

Beyond its obvious advantages, expressive writing helps people become more emotionally resilient. People who practice this on a regular basis can improve their capacity for proactive stress and anxiety management. Emotion venting, subject exploration, and time-limited writing sessions are a few of the effective strategies for emotional regulation that provide an organized method of facing and resolving difficult feelings.

Even though expressive writing is an effective way to let go of emotions, it can occasionally make one feel overwhelmed. To lessen this, creating a welcoming and secure writing place and beginning with quick sessions might help foster an atmosphere that is conducive to emotional inquiry. A kind and loving attitude to self-discovery is ensured by gradually increasing writing time as comfort levels rise.

Including expressive writing in one's daily routine can take many different forms, such as dream analysis, gratitude journals, and trauma narratives. Every exercise has a unique function and provides a customized method for attending to particular emotional requirements. For instance, Emily, a soldier with post-traumatic stress disorder, used expressive writing as a means of processing her horrific memories, which helped her on the road to healing and mental stability.

Writing that is expressive is proof of the transformational and healing power of words. It provides a methodical approach to self-reflection and emotional expression, enabling people to navigate their emotional landscapes and promoting resilience, clarity, and overall well-being. Whether dealing with ongoing stress or the fallout from terrible experiences, expressive writing provides a route to emotional release and recovery.

*Techniques for managing
your time to stop
overthinking:*

In today's fast-paced world, managing one's time is important to reduce stress and prevent overthinking. Overthinking often comes from feeling overwhelmed by tasks, deadlines, and the pressure to perform, which can significantly impact mental and physical health. By adopting strategic time management techniques, individuals can create a more balanced and fulfilling lifestyle. This content discusses various strategies to manage time efficiently, thereby minimizing stress and curbing the tendency to overthink.

Understanding Time Management and Its Importance

Time management is the art of organizing and planning how to allocate your time between different activities. It is possible for individuals to work smarter, rather than harder, in order to accomplish more in a shorter amount of time, even when time is limited and pressures are strong. This is made possible by effective time management. Effective time management leads to better efficiency and productivity, less stress, and more success in life.

Strategies for Effective Time Management

1. Setting SMART Goals

Setting Specific, Measurable, Achievable, Relevant, and Time-bound (SMART) goals is crucial for successful time management.

SMART goals provide a clear roadmap for what needs to be accomplished, making it easier to manage time and resources successfully. By setting SMART goals, people can focus their efforts on what truly matters, reducing the risk of overthinking and stress. Some of these SMART goals include: prioritizing daily tasks, limiting the use of social media, improving project deadline adherence, adopting a daily review routine, etc.

2. Prioritization

Learning to prioritize tasks based on their importance and urgency is key to managing time successfully. The Eisenhower Matrix, which categorizes tasks into four quadrants (urgent and important, important but not urgent, urgent but not important, and neither urgent nor important), can be a helpful tool in determining what tasks to focus on first.

3. Avoiding Multitasking

While multitasking might seem like an efficient way to get more done, it often leads to decreased output and increased stress. Focusing on one job at a time ensures better quality of work and reduces the chances of overthinking and making mistakes.

4. Effective Planning and Scheduling

Using a calendar or planner to schedule tasks, meetings, and deadlines can help keep track of obligations and manage time more effectively. Allocating specific time blocks for different tasks and activities can avoid overbooking and reduce stress.

5. Delegation

Not every job requires your personal attention. Identifying jobs that can be delegated to others can free up time for more critical activities. Delegation not only helps in controlling time better but also empowers others by entrusting them with responsibilities.

6. Taking Breaks

To keep working and avoid getting burned out, it's important to take breaks often. Short breaks during work can help refresh the mind, improve focus, and reduce stress, making it easier to manage time and tasks efficiently.

7. Limiting Distractions

Identifying and limiting time-wasting activities and distractions can greatly improve time management. Creating a conducive work environment, turning off unnecessary notifications, and setting limits can help one stay focused and use time more effectively.

8. Reflection and Adjustment

Regularly reviewing what was achieved against what was planned can provide insights into how effectively time is being managed. Reflecting on wins and areas for improvement allows for adjustments in strategies and techniques, ensuring continuous improvement in time management skills.

Effective time management is a critical skill that can help reduce stress and prevent overthinking. By making SMART goals, prioritizing tasks, focusing on one task at a time, successfully planning and scheduling, delegating when appropriate, taking regular breaks, limiting distractions, and regularly reflecting on and adjusting strategies, individuals can manage their time more efficiently. These strategies not only add to better productivity and success but also improve overall well-being by reducing stress and minimizing the tendency to overthink.

Setting realistic goals and assigning tasks a priority.

To simplify and elaborate on the concept of prioritizing activities and setting realistic goals as a means of managing time and inputs, let us divide the essence of effective time management into more digestible chunks, stressing critical strategies and techniques.

Understanding Time Management

Time management is really about managing your activities so that you may be as effective and productive as possible. This involves: Identifying priorities: Determine which jobs are most important and require immediate attention, just as you would sort through a mixed playlist to locate your favorite songs.

Setting realistic goals and assigning tasks a priority

Consider each objective as a single track on an album. Each should be obvious, attainable, and relevant, adding to the broader theme or goal you're going for.

Key Strategies and Techniques:

1. Eisenhower Matrix (Urgent-Important Matrix): Imagine categorizing your work into four groups that are comparable to music genres. Other tasks are urgent (requiring immediate attention),

others are vital (contributing considerably to your goals), and others may be less so. This matrix helps you focus on what is genuinely important.

2. To-Do Lists: Writing down your tasks is similar to drafting a setlist for a concert. It allows you to see what comes next and keeps you focused on the upcoming performance.

3. The Pomodoro Technique: This entails working in short, focused bursts (similar to playing a song), followed by a brief rest period. It's a

technique to keep your energy up and your mind focused.

4. Time Blocking: Set aside specified blocks of time for separate tasks, similar to scheduling studio time to record different parts of a piece. This ensures that each activity receives concentrated attention without overlap.

5. The ABCDE Method: Prioritize your chores by marking them A (most important) through E (eliminate). It's similar to organizing your music

library by favorites, ensuring you listen to the greatest songs first.

Implementing Time Management.

Use planning tools: Use tools that appeal to you, whether they are digital apps or physical planners, just like you would choose between digital or vinyl records for music playing.

Get Organized. Keep your workplace and schedule organized, much like a musician organizes their instruments and sheet music for convenient access during a performance.

Manage distractions: Identify and reduce time-wasting activities. If social media is a source of distraction for you, impose a curfew like you would on a school night.

Effective time management is similar to composing and playing music. By establishing your priorities, creating realistic goals, and implementing the appropriate strategies and approaches, you may create a productivity symphony. Like in music, where practice makes perfect, the key to mastering time management is regular application and tweaking of these concepts to suit your individual rhythm and speed.

David, an entrepreneur, noticed that his overthinking was mostly due to feeling overwhelmed by his constant to-do list. He opted to embrace the Eisenhower Matrix, a time management tool that helped him prioritize work based on urgency and importance. This simple yet successful method allowed David to focus on what was genuinely important, decreasing his temptation to overthink decisions. As a result, his firm prospered, and he found more time for personal development and relaxation. David's experience highlights how effective time and resource management may alleviate overthinking.

Chapter 6

How to Achieve Zen Instantly

Zen, stemming from Mahayana Buddhism, is a tradition stressing meditation and intuition rather than detailed doctrinal understanding, aiming for deep insight into one's nature and the essence of existence. In simplest terms, Zen is about attaining serenity and understanding via meditation, focusing on the present moment, and experiencing life directly rather than through preconceived notions and instructions.

Origins and Development

Zen's roots stretch back to China some 1,500 years ago, known as Ch'an, which is the Chinese pronunciation of Dhyana, a Sanskrit term for meditation. Zen found its way to Japan, Korea (where it's called Seon), and Vietnam (known as Thien), becoming important to these societies. The major character in Zen's creation is Bodhidharma, called the First Patriarch of Zen in China, tying the practice directly to the Buddha and emphasizing a lineage of teachers as vital to its legacy.

Core Principles

Zen is characterized by a few essential principles:

Direct Transmission: Zen highlights the importance of face-to-face transmission of teachings, favoring the direct interaction between master and student over written writings.

No Dependence on teachings: While not fully rejecting Buddhist teachings,

Zen argues for direct experience and personal insight as the way to enlightenment.

Seeing into One's Nature: The ultimate goal in Zen is to attain a deep, intuitive insight into one's true nature and the nature of reality.

The immediate relaxation methods to stop overthinking

To effectively combat overthinking and bring instant relief, employing quick relaxation techniques can be incredibly beneficial. Here are several methods, drawn from a variety of sources, intended to reduce stress and enhance your well-being promptly:

1. Deep Breathing

Deep breathing is a simple yet powerful relaxation technique that includes taking slow, deep breaths to reduce stress levels. It can be performed almost anywhere and helps to disengage the mind from distracting thoughts, promoting a state of calmness.

2. Progressive Muscle Relaxation

This method involves tensing and then relaxing different muscle groups in the body, which can help you become more aware of physical sensations and aid in releasing tension. Starting from your feet and working your way up to your face can systematically lower stress.

3. Body Scan Meditation

Body scan meditation focuses attention on different parts of the body, one at a time, without actively trying to change anything. Simply watching the sensations in each part of the body can lead to a state of deep relaxation and mindfulness.

4. Guided Imagery

Using guided imagery, you can make up calming scenes in your mind to help you relax and focus. This method involves visualizing a peaceful setting and using sensory details to deepen the relaxation experience.

5. Mindfulness Meditation

Sitting comfortably and focusing on your breathing while bringing your mind's attention to the present without drifting into worries about the past or future, can help alleviate anxiety, sadness, and pain. This exercise encourages a state of mindfulness that can reduce stress.

6. Yoga, Tai Chi, and Qigong

These practices combine rhythmic breathing with a number of postures or flowing movements, giving a mental focus that can help distract from racing thoughts. They also improve flexibility and balance, contributing to overall stress reduction.

7. Repetitive Prayer

For those who find spirituality important, quietly repeating a prayer or phrase while practicing breath focus can be a comforting and relaxing technique.

8. Simple Visualization Exercise

Creating a mental picture of a peaceful and happy place can help focus the mind and bring relaxation.

Engaging all senses in this visualization strengthens the effect, making it a powerful tool against stress.

9. Quick Muscle Relaxation

This includes tensing and then relaxing each muscle group in turn, which can quickly relieve tension. Focusing on the breath while doing this can improve relaxation.

10. Cued Relaxation

After mastering some relaxation exercises, using a 'cue' throughout the day can tell you to relax your muscles, check your breathing, and lower stress levels on the spot. Incorporating these techniques into your daily routine, even if just for a few minutes at a time, can provide a reserve of inner calm and greatly reduce the impact of stress and overthinking on your life. Remember, the key to benefiting from these methods is regular practice and finding the ones that best suit your preferences and lifestyle.

The benefits of breathing techniques and visualization for calming the mind

Breathing exercises and visualization are powerful tools for gaining mental calm and reducing stress. These techniques are not only accessible and cost-effective but also backed by scientific study and evidence.

Breathing Exercises

Breathing exercises, particularly deep breathing or diaphragmatic breathing, have been shown to have a positive effect on various factors like stress, anxiety, and negative affect. Deep breathing involves slow, deep inhalations through the nose, which allows more oxygen to enter the body and promote relaxation. This type of breathing stimulates the parasympathetic nervous system, which is responsible for the body's rest and digest reaction, thereby reducing stress and anxiety levels.

Studies have proven that deep breathing exercises can enhance blood oxygen levels, stimulate the vagus nerve, and promote a state of calmness. For instance, an experiment performed in China with 40 healthy participants found that over the course of deep breathing treatment, participants experienced increased sustained attention and decreased negative affect and cortisol levels.Another study with presurgical patients showed that deep breathing, along with lavender aromatherapy, greatly reduced preoperative anxiety in approximately 40% of the patients.

Visualization

Visualization, or guided imagery, is another effective method for achieving mental calm. It includes creating mental images or scenarios that are calming or beneficial to the person. This exercise can help in reducing stress, anxiety, and even pain. Visualization works by engaging the brain in a focused and positive way, diverting attention from worry and negative thoughts.

Research has found that guided imagery can significantly reduce death anxiety among nurses working in COVID-19 intensive care units, highlighting its usefulness in high-stress settings [0]. Visualization exercises often involve imagining a peaceful scene, such as a beach or a forest, and focusing on the sensory experiences connected with that scene (e.g., the sound of waves and the smell of trees) to deepen the relaxation effect.

Integrating Breathing Exercises and Visualization

Integrating breathing exercises with visualization can amplify the stress-relieving effects of both practices. For example, one can perform deep breathing while simultaneously picturing a calming color or scene. This combination involves both the body and mind in relaxation, leading to a more profound state of calmness.

The effectiveness of these techniques is supported by scientific studies. A study provided evidence of the benefits of progressive muscle relaxation (PMR), deep breathing, and guided imagery for stress relaxation, proving their positive effect on both psychological and physiological states of relaxation. It's important to note that while all three methods caused relaxation, PMR and guided imagery were found to have a more robust effect on physiological relaxation compared to deep breathing alone.

Breathing techniques and visualization are potent tools for managing stress and achieving mental calm. They are easy to practice, require no special tools, and can be done almost anywhere. By incorporating these techniques into daily routines, people can greatly improve their mental well-being, reduce stress levels, and enhance their quality of life. The scientific evidence supporting these practices underscores their worth as part of a holistic approach to stress management and mental health.

Chapter 7

Newfound Awareness-
Based Attitudes

Clarity, engagement, and a profound comprehension of the audience's requirements and preferences are all necessary components in the process of developing content that will resonate with your audience. It is essential to express complicated concepts in a way that is not only understandable but also compelling, regardless of whether you are speaking to novices or seasoned professionals. To ensure that your message not only reaches your audience but also has an influence on them in a meaningful way, here is how to strengthen your approach.

A Comprehension of Your Target Audience

When it comes to writing that has an impact, having a solid grasp of your audience is the cornerstone. They are captivated by what? On what basis do they bring their expertise to the table? By providing responses to these questions, you will be able to modify your content in a manner that is immediately relevant to the particular interests and degree of comprehension of the audience. An example of this would be that novices in a certain field might value analogies and straightforward explanations more than

Forming attitudes that
support presence and
awareness:

Developing attitudes that enhance mindfulness and presence includes building a mental environment where awareness and acceptance are at the forefront. Mindfulness, a practice with roots in ancient Buddhist teachings, has transcended its origins to become a vital tool for increasing mental and emotional resilience in contemporary society. This topic addresses the value of mindfulness and how particular attitudes might strengthen its practice, ultimately leading to a more present and fulfilling existence.

The Core Attitudes of Mindfulness Acknowledgment is about acknowledging and accepting things as they are. This attitude supports embracing the present moment without trying to change or reject what emerges, establishing an environment of acceptance.

Non-striving entails letting go of the drive to achieve specific results and instead focusing on being content with where we are. This mindset aids in finding fulfillment in the current moment, eliminating the persistent pursuit of future goals that frequently leads to discontent.

Equanimity refers to retaining balance and knowledge in the face of change. It teaches us to be present with change, acknowledge the impermanence of life, and handle problems with compassion and wisdom.

Self-Reliance highlights the value of self-discovery and finding truth through our experiences. This attitude produces a strong sense of authenticity and insights that match our beliefs, motivating us to trust ourselves.

Self-compassion involves treating ourselves with care and understanding, without self-blame or judgment. Cultivating self-compassion allows us to appreciate our shortcomings and builds a supportive relationship with ourselves.

Generosity, the act of giving without expectation, establishes connections and has a good influence. Practicing generosity not only benefits others but also enriches our own lives, highlighting the reciprocal nature of giving and receiving. Integrating Mindfulness into Daily Life

Mindfulness can be practiced in ordinary tasks such as eating, walking, and working. By bringing awareness to these actions, we can transform boring duties into moments of present and appreciation. For example, relishing each mouthful of a meal, experiencing the sensation of our feet contacting the ground while walking, or focusing on one job at a time during work can improve our mindfulness practice.

Mindfulness-Based Programs

Programs like Mindfulness-Based Stress Reduction (MBSR) and Mindfulness-Based Cognitive

Therapy (MBCT) offer organized techniques to increase mindfulness. These programs have demonstrated success in lowering anxiety and depression and improving overall well-being. They offer different awareness approaches, like meditation, body scans, and mindful eating, which can be integrated into daily life to manage stress and increase mental health.

Mindfulness in the Workplace

Incorporating mindfulness programs in corporate settings can lead to a more engaged and resilient workforce. These programs may include mindfulness training, meditation breaks, and group mindfulness practices, promoting a work atmosphere that promotes well-being, creativity, and productivity.

The Future of Mindfulness

As mindfulness continues to expand, emerging trends and innovations, such as technology-integrated practices and digital mindfulness resources, are making mindfulness more accessible.

However, the difficulty continues to sustain presence and awareness in the digital age, navigating distractions while creating a mindful lifestyle.

Developing attitudes that support mindfulness and presence is a transforming journey that enriches our quality of life. By embracing attitudes such as acknowledgment, non-striving, equanimity, self-reliance, self-compassion, and generosity, we can create a greater sense of awareness, resilience, and compassion. Integrating mindfulness into daily activities, participating in mindfulness-based programs, and embracing mindfulness in the workplace are practical strategies to cultivate these attitudes. As we navigate the future of mindfulness, it is crucial to remember the underlying concepts that make mindfulness a powerful tool for personal growth and well-being.

Reducing overthinking that is focused on the future by learning to live in the now

Learning to live in the moment is an important ability for avoiding future-oriented overthinking, which can cause anxiety, stress, and missed possibilities for joy and connection in the present. The approaches and ideas shared by diverse sources provide actionable measures for anybody wishing to build mindfulness and presence in their daily lives.

The Value of Present-Moment Awareness

Overthinking about the future can distract us from our current experiences, creating a cycle of perpetual worry and stress. By focusing on the current moment, we can interrupt the pattern, lowering anxiety and improving our overall well-being. Living in the present now allows us to appreciate the richness of life as it unfolds, which improves our connections with others and our capacity to focus and enjoy our everyday tasks.

Breathing exercises

Breathing exercises are an important tool for grounding oneself in the present moment. Mindful breathing entails focusing on the sensation of breath as it enters and departs the body, which can help to relax the mind and prevent overthinking. This practice can be done anywhere and at any time, making it a versatile tool for cultivating mindfulness and stress reduction.

Meditation

Meditation is another effective technique for increasing present-moment awareness. It teaches us to examine our thoughts and feelings without judgment, letting us let go of concerns about the past and future. Regular meditation practice can boost mental clarity, emotional stability, and overall well-being. Starting with just a few minutes each day can significantly improve one's ability to live more mindfully.

For individuals who prefer a more structured approach to mindfulness, Mindfulness-Based Stress Reduction provides an 8-week program that combines meditation, body awareness, and yoga to help reduce stress and promote present-moment awareness. Jon Kabat-Zinn developed MBSR, which has been demonstrated to offer a variety of advantages, including reduced anxiety and depression symptoms, improved focus, and improved emotional control.

Journaling

Journaling is a reflective exercise that can help us become more aware of our thoughts and feelings, making it simpler to identify when we are overthinking the future. Free writing or journal prompts can help us slow down our thoughts and focus more on the present moment, thus promoting the development of mindfulness and presence.

Savoring

To overcome the habit of worrying about the future, try relishing the present moment. This entails taking the time to completely interact with and enjoy current experiences, such as savoring a meal, having a conversation, or admiring nature. By focusing on our senses and the delight in everyday events, we may educate our minds to be more present.

Engagement and Flow

Engaging fully in activities can also assist in preventing overthinking by fostering a state of flow in which one is completely immersed in what they are doing. Setting specific goals and choosing activities that fit our ability level might help us achieve this state, making it simpler to lose track of time and worry about the future. Flow activities boost not only our quality of life but also our performance and creativity.

Acceptance and Nonresistance

Finally, learning to embrace discomfort rather than avoid it might assist in controlling overthinking.

Acceptance of our current emotions and experiences, rather than attempting to modify or reject them, can help to alleviate the tension that comes with resisting reality. This technique promotes a more tranquil and welcoming mindset, which is favorable to living in the present moment.

Implementing these activities in daily life can considerably increase one's ability to live in the present moment, lessening the inclination to overthink the future. Individuals can improve their mental and emotional well-being by practicing mindfulness through breathing exercises, meditation, MBSR, journaling, savoring, flow activities, and acceptance.

Chapter 8

Building a Support System

In the complicated tapestry of human existence, the threads of social ties and community build a pattern of support and resilience, which is essential for navigating the labyrinth of our thoughts, particularly when they spiral into overthinking. The dance of social connection is essential for regulating the tornado of our minds, providing a haven of understanding, empathy, and shared experiences.

Symphony of Social Connections

Consider the human psyche to be a vast ocean with waves that are both peaceful and turbulent. When these waves threaten to become a storm of overthinking, the anchor of social relationships is crucial. Engaging with others, sharing laughter, and even the mere act of listening can lift our spirits, similar to how a harmonic symphony soothes the soul. This encounter serves as a salve, raising us from the depths of our thoughts and grounding us in the present.

The alchemy of altruism

Altruism, or unselfish concern for the well-being of others, is like a powerful elixir for the spirit. When we move outside of ourselves to help others, we engage in a transforming process. This act of giving, with no hope of recompense, not only strengthens the recipient but also benefits the donor. It serves as a reminder of our common humanity, instilling thankfulness and perspective that can help to lighten the burden of our own problems and overthinking.

Nurturing Social Gardens

For those who are ensnared by the thorns of overthinking, creating a garden of social ties can be a step toward freedom. Starting conversations, joining groups that share our interests, and developing constructive relationships are like planting seeds of support that can blossom into a rich oasis of comfort and understanding. However, just like in any garden, boundaries are necessary to keep this space from becoming a source of further stress. Embracing acceptance and commitment.

When navigating the social waters, it is critical to recognize and accept any waves of uneasiness that may develop. Acceptance and Commitment Therapy (ACT) provides a compass for this journey, enabling us to accept our ideas and feelings with openness and compassion. This technique promotes a harmonious relationship with our inner selves, allowing us to communicate more fully and truthfully with others.

Seeking professional beacons.

Recognizing when to seek professional aid demonstrates strength and self-awareness. Overthinking, when it becomes a storm in our daily lives, needs the assistance of mental health professionals. Cognitive-behavioral therapy (CBT) and Mindfulness-

Based Stress Reduction (MBSR) are two therapies that can help you navigate through the fog of rumination and find a brighter sky.

Creating a support system is analogous to building a bridge across the turbulent waters of overthinking. It's about making connections that provide comfort, understanding, and a sense of belonging. Through social connection, charity, and professional direction, we can return to the shore, where thoughts are merely ripples on the surface of a deeper, more serene sea of consciousness.

The importance of social interaction and community in managing overthinking

The value of social connection and community in overcoming overthinking cannot be emphasized. Social engagement has a significant impact on our mental health since it affects hormone balance. Participating in social activities, in particular, can boost oxytocin levels, a hormone that reduces anxiety while increasing our sense of attachment and connection to others. This hormone boost not only makes us feel less anxious but also more confident in our capacity to cope with challenges, which perpetuates a loop of seeking additional social support.

Furthermore, socialization directs our attention outward, offering momentary relief from personal tension and fostering a sense of belonging and inclusion. This external attention can be especially useful for people who overthink since it allows them to temporarily disconnect from their internal monologue and engage with others. Sharing concerns and feelings with others can reduce stress and improve mood, resulting in a more meaningful and purposeful life.

Altruism, or the act of assisting others without expecting anything in return, is another effective method for controlling overthinking. Altruistic activities increase neurotransmitters associated with happy emotions, reducing anxiety and concern. This outward emphasis not only relieves tension but also provides a new perspective on one's own gifts, encouraging thankfulness and decreasing the desire for worldly items. Furthermore, compassion has been connected to better life adjustment, significance, relationship happiness, and physical wellness.

For people who struggle with overthinking, actively seeking out social contacts can be a helpful tactic.

Starting conversations, joining groups or programs, and building positive relationships can help to relieve stress. It is critical, however, to strike a balance and establish boundaries to ensure that socialization is a source of comfort rather than stress.

Acceptance and Commitment Therapy (ACT) provides effective approaches for dealing with anxiety that may arise during social encounters. One such strategy is to acknowledge and appreciate your mind for its protective intentions, even if it results in overthinking or social anxiety. This technique promotes a gentler, more accepting attitude toward oneself and one's experiences, allowing for a better interaction with one's ideas and feelings.

Developing social relationships and engaging in altruistic activities can be effective in managing overthinking. These activities not only provide instant stress relief but also help to foster a stronger feeling of purpose and well-being.

Furthermore, using ACT strategies can help people overcome the obstacles of social anxiety, encouraging a more caring and welcoming perspective.

How to seek help and when to consider professional assistance

Seeking aid and considering professional help to reduce overthinking is an important step for anyone who is stuck in a cycle of rumination and anxious thoughts. Overthinking can take many forms, including ruminating on the past, fretting about the future, or obsessing over decisions and their possible effects. While it is natural to experience some amount of reflection and anxiety, when these thoughts become excessive, they can cause severe anguish and impair one's ability to operate well in everyday life.

Knowing when to seek help.

The first step in dealing with overthinking is to recognize when it has become a problem. Overthinking can have negative effects on your well-being, such as difficulty making decisions owing to anxiety about making the wrong choice.

Symptoms may include: - Constant mental replay or analysis - Anxiety or tension over uncontrollable events - And difficulty sleeping due to racing thoughts.

Feeling mentally fatigued but unable to interrupt the cycle of thoughts.

When overthinking interferes with your daily tasks, relationships, or overall mental health, it's time to seek help.

Self-help Strategies.

Before seeking professional treatment, you might attempt the following self-help strategies:

Accept or Deny Your Thoughts: Understand that not every thought requires your attention or reply. Learn to observe them without engaging.

Meditation and mindfulness: Practices such as meditation can help you focus your attention and lessen the impact of distracting ideas. Mindfulness encourages you to live in the present moment, eliminating worry about the future and sorrow about the past.

Physical Exercise: Physical activity helps divert you from overthinking and release endorphins, which boost your mood.

- Journaling: Writing down your thoughts can help you organize and perceive them in a new light, making it easier to let go of useless ruminating.

Professional assistance.

If self-help measures are ineffective in managing your overthinking, it may be necessary to seek professional treatment. Mental health specialists, such as therapists or counselors, can help you overcome your overthinking habits. They can provide:

Cognitive-Behavioral Therapy (CBT): CBT is beneficial in treating overthinking because it helps people identify and fight harmful thought patterns, replacing them with more realistic and positive ones.

Mindfulness-Based Stress Reduction (MBSR): MBSR uses mindfulness meditation to relieve stress and anxiety, which might be useful for people who overthink.

Support Groups: Joining a support group can help you feel more connected and understood, as well as providing strategies that others have found useful.

When to Seek Professional Help.

Seek professional help if overthinking causes considerable distress or impairment in social, occupational, or other vital areas of functioning.

Overthinking is causing you to experience symptoms of anxiety, sadness, or other mental health difficulties.

Self-help efforts have not resulted in improvement.

It's critical to remember that requesting help is an indication of strength, not weakness. Mental health professionals are educated to offer the support and resources required to effectively manage overthinking. Professional help, whether in the form of therapy, medicine, or a combination of techniques, can significantly enhance your capacity to control your thoughts and quality of life.

Chapter 9

Accepting
Unpredictability

In the vast expanse of life's journey, the winds of uncertainty are ever-present, whispering of unknown futures and paths yet to be found. Embracing this uncertainty, rather than attempting to outmaneuver it with exhaustive analysis, can change our experience of life from one of apprehension to one of adventure and growth. Here, we study methods to navigate the uncharted waters of the unknown with grace and resilience.

Embracing the Inevitable Dance of Uncertainty

Life, in its infinite complexity, gives no guarantees, save for the promise of unpredictability. Recognizing uncertainty as an inherent feature of existence liberates us from the futile pursuit of absolute control. This acceptance invites us to live more fully in the present, engaging with life as it happens, rather than being ensnared by the endless "what-ifs"that lie beyond our grasp.

Steering Through the Storm with Agency

In the huge ocean of life's uncertainties, our focus becomes our rudder. By directing our attention to the elements within our reach—the actions we can take, the choices we can make—we reclaim our power. This shift from a passive to an active stance empowers us to navigate through uncertainty with purpose and determination, charting a path through the waters of the unknown with the actions we can control.

Questioning the Quest for Certainty

The craving for certainty, often based on fear, can be a cage that confines us to the familiar, inhibiting growth and exploration. By challenging this need, we open ourselves to the possibilities that uncertainty brings—the chances for learning, the potential for surprise, and the joy of discovery. This reframe transforms uncertainty from a source of anxiety to a catalyst for growth and evolution.

Curating Our Consumption

In our quest for understanding, it's easy to become overwhelmed by the deluge of knowledge that bombards us daily. Recognizing when to step back, to limit our intake of news and social media, can help keep our equilibrium. By choosing when and how we interact with the world's narratives, we protect our peace and avoid the amplification of our anxieties.

Anchoring in the Now

Mindfulness, the art of being fully present, gives a sanctuary from the storms of uncertainty. Through practices like meditation, deep breathing, and yoga, we can ground ourselves in the moment, finding calm and clarity amidst the chaos. This presence helps us to meet uncertainty not as a foe to be vanquished but as a companion on our journey, teaching us to flow with life's ever-changing tides.

Cultivating a Circle of Support

No one is an island, and in times of uncertainty, the value of a supportive group becomes immeasurable. Reaching out, and sharing our fears and hopes, can lighten our burdens and broaden our views. This shared journey through the unknown strengthens our bonds and reminds us that, though the road may be uncertain, we do not walk it alone.

Nurturing Ourselves

Self-care is our lifeline in managing uncertainty. By prioritizing our well-being—through exercise, diet, rest, and hobbies—we build resilience against the stressors of the unknown. This foundation of self-care equips us to face uncertainty not as a danger but as an adventure, with power and vitality.

There are times when the waves of uncertainty threaten to overwhelm us when the strategies we've applied are not enough to quell the storm. In these times, reaching out for professional support can be a beacon of hope, guiding us back to calmer waters.

In embracing uncertainty, we start on a journey of growth, discovery, and resilience. By accepting the unknown as an integral part of life, focusing on what we can control, and nurturing ourselves and our relationships, we can navigate the unpredictable currents of existence with grace and courage. In the dance with uncertainty, we find not only challenges but also opportunities—for in the heart of the unknown lie the seeds of

possibility, waiting to be found.

Techniques for handling the unfamiliar without becoming too analytical

Dealing with the unknown and the uncertainties that come with it may be a substantial source of stress and anxiety for many people. Overthinking alternative outcomes or scenarios typically leads to further worry rather than delivering any genuine solutions. However, there are effective ways that can aid in regulating these sentiments and creating a more resilient approach towards uncertainty.

1. Accept Uncertainty as a Part of Life

Understanding and accepting that uncertainty is an intrinsic aspect of life can be freeing. It permits you to change your focus from trying to foresee or control the future to dealing with present realities more effectively. Recognize that no matter how much you plan, you can never account for every outcome. Accepting this helps diminish the need for certainty and alleviates the tension that comes with trying to anticipate the future.

2. Focus on What You Can Control

Concentrate on actions and decisions within your control rather than fretting about those that aren't. This shift in emphasis can energize you and create a sense of agency. For example, while you may not be able to influence the outcome of a job application, you can control how well you prepare for an interview or how many applications you submit. Focusing on these controllable characteristics can lead to more productive behaviors and less rumination.

3. Challenge Your Need for Certainty

Question the requirement of having assurance in every element of life. Often, the urge for certainty is fueled by fear of the unknown or fear of making mistakes. By overcoming these worries and recognizing that uncertainty can lead to growth, opportunity, and new experiences, you can begin to perceive uncertainty in a more positive manner. Consider the merits and downsides of certainty, and reflect on situations when an unexpected conclusion led to a positive surprise.

4. Limit Exposure to News and Information Overload

Constantly seeking information or updates, especially in today's digital age, can aggravate worry and tension. Limit your exposure to news and social media, particularly outlets that focus on worst-case scenarios or speculative material. Instead, assign particular intervals for updates and use credible sources to avoid information overload.

5. Practice Mindfulness and Present Moment Awareness

Mindfulness exercises can help you stay anchored in the current moment, lowering anxieties about the future. By focusing on the here and now, you can escape the pattern of overthinking and catastrophizing about what might happen. Mindfulness methods, such as meditation, deep breathing, or yoga, can help lower stress and improve your overall well-being.

6. Build a Support System

Having a solid support system can bring comfort and stability during times of uncertainty. Reach out to friends, relatives, or support groups to discuss your experiences and worries. Often, merely talking about your issues can provide relief and offer new views. Remember, requesting support is a sign of strength, not weakness.

7. Engage in Self-Care

Maintaining healthy routines and engaging in activities that enhance well-being are vital during times of stress. Exercise, eat healthily, get adequate sleep, and make time for hobbies or activities that offer you joy. Prioritizing self-care can assist in regulating stress levels and boost your resilience against the challenges offered by uncertainty.

8. Seek Professional Help When Needed

If emotions of anxiety or tension become excessive or interfere with your daily life, consider seeking professional treatment. A mental health professional can offer techniques and resources to manage overthinking and provide assistance in overcoming uncertainty.

While the unknown can be a cause of anxiety, adopting these

tactics can help you negotiate ambiguity with greater confidence and less stress. By focusing on what you can control, recognizing uncertainty as a part of life, and taking care of your mental health, you may reduce overthinking and live a more balanced and satisfying life.

Facing uncertainty and finding calmness in it

Learning to accept and find serenity in uncertainty is an essential ability for preserving mental and emotional health in an unpredictable world. Here are some ideas from many sources that can help you grow acceptance and tranquility in the midst of uncertainty.

1. Recognize Uncertainty as Part of Life.

Understand and embrace that uncertainty is a natural and inescapable part of life. We may apply this acceptance to bigger elements of our lives, just as we do with daily uncertainties like traffic or food safety. Recognizing that some level of uncertainty and unpredictability is inherent in many of our daily activities can help us become more accepting of uncertainty in other areas.

2. Identify and reduce uncertainty triggers.

Be conscious of what causes your feelings of uncertainty. External variables, such as excessive media intake or conversations with nervous people, can exacerbate your own concerns and uncertainty. By identifying these triggers, you may minimize your exposure to them, lowering your overall anxiety levels.

3. Allow yourself to be uncertain.

Instead of opposing or attempting to control the uncontrollable, let yourself feel the discomfort associated with uncertainty. Recognizing and experiencing your feelings without judgment will help them pass faster. Deep breathing and meditation are two techniques that can help you stay in the present moment and reduce the discomfort that uncertainty causes.

4. Redirect Your Attention to the Present

Worrying about the future simply exacerbates feelings of uncertainty and can lead to a loss of hope. Instead, focus on the present moment. Mindfulness activities can help you shift your focus from future anxieties to the present moment, increasing your appreciation for it and calming your mind.

5. Acceptance Does Not Mean Inaction.

Accepting uncertainty should not indicate apathy or resignation. It is nevertheless beneficial to plan for the future while accepting that you cannot predict or control every result. Acceptance allows you to deal with current realities more effectively, without the added burden of predicting every conceivable outcome.

6. Accept the Lessons of Uncertainty.

Negative experiences and uncertainty can be effective teachers. They teach resilience, adaptability, and the finding of inner strength. Accepting uncertainty as an opportunity for progress can change your viewpoint, allowing you to perceive obstacles as opportunities to learn and grow.

7. Practice self-compassion and mindfulness.

Be compassionate to yourself while you're feeling uncertain.

Practicing self-compassion and mindfulness can help you negotiate these times with grace and patience. Mindfulness, in particular, can help you develop a stronger connection with yourself by quieting the cacophony in your mind and making you more open to new ideas and paths.

8. Seek Support

Do not hesitate to seek help from friends, family, or experts. Sharing your emotions and experiences with others can bring comfort and new perspectives. Remember that asking for help is a show of strength and a crucial step toward better uncertainty management.

Finding serenity in uncertainty entails accepting life's inherent unpredictability, limiting exposure to triggers, focusing on the present, and welcoming the opportunities for growth that uncertainty presents. Integrating these tactics into your daily life can help you develop a more tranquil and resilient mindset in the face of the unknown.

Lily, a financial analyst, suffered ongoing concern over the unpredictable nature of the stock market. Her turning moment came when she attended a course on embracing uncertainty. She learned to focus on what she could control, such as her research and analysis processes, rather than the outcomes. Lily also started practicing mindfulness to stay grounded in the present moment. These improvements helped her embrace the inherent uncertainty of her career, considerably lowering her overthinking and anxiety. Lily's tale highlights the significance of accepting uncertainty as a part of life and finding serenity within it.

Chapter 10

Moving On Without Thinking Too Much

Overanalyzing life is a road that leads to mental captivity. Let go and move forward. It's about letting go of the constant impulse to scrutinize every little detail and bravely facing the unknown.

Fundamentally, trusting oneself and the universe is the key to going on without overanalyzing. It's admitting that not every choice has to be examined in great detail and examined till it causes paralysis. Rather, it's about being open to the possibilities that lay ahead and taking measured chances.

Acceptance is essential to moving on without second-guessing yourself. acceptance of the past, including ruined relationships, squandered opportunities, and errors in judgment. Relying too much on the past just keeps us stuck in a rut. We free ourselves to concentrate on the here and now and the things we can do to influence the future by accepting the things that cannot be altered.

Another essential element of moving on without overanalyzing is forgiveness. This includes pardoning those who may have harmed us as well as pardoning ourselves for previous transgressions. Keeping grudges or resentments close to our hearts just makes things heavier and keeps us from progressing. Forgiveness frees us from the emotional burden that prevents us from moving forward and makes room for development and recovery.

One of the hardest parts of moving on without overanalyzing is probably letting go of control. Although it's only human nature to want to be in charge of everything in our lives, there are certain things that are just out of our hands. For inner peace and contentment, it is imperative to learn to let go and trust that life will develop as it should.

Remaining mindful is essential to moving past overanalyzing. We can learn to notice our thoughts and feelings objectively and without bias by engaging in mindfulness practices. This enables us to break free from unfavorable mental habits and develop improved perspective and clarity.

Another effective strategy for moving on without second-guessing is to cultivate thankfulness. By concentrating on our blessings, we turn our attention from our anxieties and fears to the abundance that is all around us. Gratitude reminds us of the wonder and beauty present in every moment and has the ability to change the way we view life.

Accepting uncertainty is necessary to move on without overanalyzing. It is impossible to control or foresee every occurrence in life because uncertainty is a natural part of life. We might choose to view the unknown as a chance for adventure and personal development rather than something to be afraid of.

Accepting uncertainty enables us to bravely and curiously enter the unknown rather than retreating out of fear.

Overcoming overthinking and moving on with life is a path of empowerment and self-discovery. It's about accepting the present, letting go of the past, and having faith in the seemingly endless possibilities of the future. We can break free from the trap of overthinking and live more completely in the present moment by engaging in practices of acceptance, forgiveness, mindfulness, gratitude, and embracing ambiguity.

Support and direction to maintain progress and avoid relapsing

To stop overthinking and make progress on your path to mental well-being, you must implement tactics that prevent you from falling back into old thought habits. Overthinking frequently results in a cycle of negative thinking, anxiety, and stress, which can impede your progress. Here are some encouraging and guiding recommendations to help you continue your progress and avoid relapse.

1. Recognize early warning signs: Recognize that relapse is a process, not an event. Identifying early warning indicators, such as increased tension, worry, or a return to old thought patterns, can help you take action before you completely relapse into overthinking.

2. Develop Healthy Coping Skills: Provide yourself with a variety of coping techniques for dealing with stress and anxiety. Mindfulness meditation, deep breathing exercises, and progressive muscle relaxation can all help you calm down and stop overthinking.

3. Challenge Negative Thoughts:

Use cognitive-behavioral tools to confront and alter negative thought patterns. When you find yourself overthinking, consider what evidence supports and opposes your views.

This can help you see situations more clearly and lessen worry.

4. Maintain a Balanced Lifestyle: Stress reduction is essential for preventing recurrence. Maintain a balanced lifestyle that includes physical activity, enough rest, nutritious nutrition, and time for relaxation and enjoyment. Avoiding becoming overly hungry, angry, lonely, or tired (HALT) can also aid in stress management and prevent overthinking.

5. Create a Support Network: Surround yourself with sympathetic friends and family, or join a support group to share your experiences and ideas for managing to overthink. Knowing you are not alone in your challenges can be reassuring and encouraging.

6. Set Realistic Goals:

Set attainable goals for yourself and appreciate your accomplishments. Recognizing your accomplishments, no matter how minor, can raise your confidence and inspire you to keep working toward your mental health.

7. Practice Self-Compassion:

Be kind to yourself and understand that progress takes time. If you have a setback, do not be too hard on yourself. Instead, use it as an opportunity to learn and improve your coping skills.

8. Seek Professional Help if Needed: If you're having trouble managing your overthinking on your own, talk to a mental health professional. They can offer specific techniques and

assistance to help you continue your progress and avoid relapse.

Remember that preventing a relapse into overthinking is a continuous process that demands patience, effort, and perseverance. By implementing these tactics, you will be able to maintain your progress, better manage stress and anxiety, and continue your journey to mental wellness.

Develop a Growth Mentality

As we end our journey through the pages of "You can quit Overthinking," we come to a critical chapter that encompasses the core of transformation and growth: "Develop a Growth Mentality."This final chapter is not only a review of what has been addressed but a beacon of light directing us toward a future where overthinking does not hold us back from realizing our highest potential. It's about embracing the power within ourselves to build a mindset that thrives on difficulties, learns from setbacks, and consistently seeks growth.

Embrace Challenges with Open Arms

The first step in building a growth mentality is to regard challenges not as insurmountable hurdles but as opportunities for learning and growth. When we adjust our perspective to see challenges as puzzles to be solved, we empower ourselves to tackle them with interest and drive. This mindset drives us to stretch beyond our current limits and discover new qualities within ourselves.

Learn from Failure

Failure is an inevitable part of the journey towards growth. However, it's not the failure itself that defines us, but how we respond to it. By reimagining failure as a stepping stone to success, we may extract essential lessons from our losses and use them to construct a path forward. This method builds resilience and guarantees that we remain devoted to our goals, even in the face of hardship.

Cultivate Persistence

Persistence is the gasoline that propels the motor of growth. It is about accepting the discomfort of the unknown and pushing through hurdles with unrelenting commitment. By committing to our goals and refusing to give up, we gain the resilience necessary to traverse the ups and downs of personal and professional development.

Seek and Utilize Feedback Constructively

Feedback is a great tool for progress, delivering insights that can help us adjust our approach and enhance our talents. By actively seeking out constructive criticism and being open to learning from it, we may find areas for development and make genuine progress towards our aims.

Surround Yourself with Growth-Minded Individuals

The company we keep can considerably influence our thoughts and attitudes. Surrounding oneself with persons who reflect a growth mentality can inspire and drive us to embrace difficulties, learn from failures, and continue in the face of adversity. Their tenacity and optimistic outlook can serve as a daily reminder of the potential of a growth mindset.

Celebrate Every Step Forward

Recognizing and applauding our success, no matter how tiny, is vital for keeping motivation and reinforcing a growth mentality. By praising the effort and dedication that goes into completing each milestone, we remind ourselves of the value of persistence and the joy of learning.

Let us carry on the lessons gained and the strategies presented. Developing a development mentality is a journey that needs patience, effort, and a willingness to welcome change. By adopting this mentality, we may overcome the barriers of overthinking and release our full potential, ready to meet the difficulties and possibilities that lie ahead with confidence and resilience.